The Ketogenic Diet Cookbook

73 Easy Recipes for Rapid Fat Loss, Laser Sharp Focus and a Better Life (Lose up to a Pound a Day! Includes Over 73 Recipes, and 73 Tips to Lose Weight & Regain Energy

Michelle Jones

The following eBook is reproduced below with the goal of providing information that is as accurate and as reliable as possible. Regardless, purchasing this eBook can be seen as consent to the fact that both the publisher and the author of this book are in no way experts on the topics discussed within, and that any recommendations or suggestions made herein are for entertainment purposes only. Professionals should be consulted as needed before undertaking any of the action endorsed herein.

This declaration is deemed fair and valid by both the American Bar Association and the Committee of Publishers Association and is legally binding throughout the United States.

Furthermore, the transmission, duplication or reproduction of any of the following work, including precise information, will be considered an illegal act, irrespective whether it is done electronically or in print. The legality extends to creating a secondary or tertiary copy of the work or a recorded copy and is only allowed with express written consent of the Publisher. All additional rights are reserved.

The information in the following pages is broadly considered to be a truthful and accurate account of facts, and as such any inattention, use or misuse of the information in question by the reader will render any resulting actions solely under their purview. There are no scenarios in which the publisher or the original author of this work can be in any fashion deemed liable for any hardship or damages that may befall them after undertaking information described herein.

Additionally, the information found on the following pages is intended for informational purposes only and should thus be considered, universal. As befitting its nature, the information presented is without assurance regarding its continued validity or interim quality. Trademarks that are mentioned are done without written consent and can in no way be considered an endorsement from the trademark holder.

Table of Contents

Introduction

Congratulations on downloading your personal copy of *The Ketogenic Diet Cookbook*. Thank you for doing so.

The following chapters will give you information about the ketogenic diet and plenty of recipes to help you get started with your new life.

There are plenty of books on this subject on the market, thanks again for choosing this one! Every effort was made to ensure it is full of as much useful information as possible. Please enjoy!

Congratulations on downloading your personal copy of *The Ketogenic Diet Cookbook*. Thank you for doing so.

What is the Ketogenic Diet?

The ketogenic diet is very low in carbs but high in fats. It will allow your body to learn to stop using carbs for energy and start breaking down the fats in your body and turning them into ketones to be used as fuel.
Your body goes into ketosis every day. You are able to eat what you want within reason. Your body has the ability to adapt and process different nutrients to be used as fuel. Everyone's body needs fuel to be able to function. The body will use proteins, fats, and carbohydrates. By consuming a diet low in carbs and high in fats will increase this process. Your body's reaction is normal and totally safe.

Every time you eat huge amounts of proteins and carbs, the body turns them into glucose. Glucose then turns it into ATP. We need this fuel to do our normal activities and help support our bodies.

If you starve your body from glucose for fuel, several different things are going to happen:

Lipogenesis: occurs when the muscles and liver have excess glycogen. Any extra gets stored as fat.

Glycogenesis: occurs when excess glucose gets turned into glycogen and stores it in the liver and muscles. The energy we use every day will get stored as glycogen.

Ketosis: happens when the body doesn't have any glycogen or glucose to use.

When you sleep, the body will build fat and create ketones. This happens because you don't have access to food.

When the body makes ketones, it starts to break down fats. This creates fatty acids that get burned by the liver. This process is called beta-oxidation. This is what makes ketones. These will be used for fuel by the muscles and brain.

To make this a bit easier to understand, if the body doesn't have any glucose or glycogen, ketosis starts and the body begins to use all the fat that has been stored in the body for energy.

Ketosis works when fats are broken down in the liver, and fatty acids and glycerol gets released. The fatty acids are broken down further in ketogenesis. This will create a process that is called acetoacetate.

With time, your body begins to expel fewer ketone bodies. You will think that ketosis is slowing down, but this isn't true. Your brain burns it as fuel, too. The body gives the brain the right amount of glucose to be used as energy.

Your body needs glucose to remain healthy. It just doesn't need as much as we think it does. Your body doesn't need carbs for fuel. The liver makes sure that it has enough glucose in the blood to keep your body healthy.

Too much protein gets turned into glucose and therefore can be dangerous to this diet and can kick you out of ketosis.

Recipes

Breakfast
Turmeric Vanilla Oatmeal

If you love oatmeal, this is a great substitute. This delicious savory oatmeal can be eaten cold. If you prefer warm oatmeal, just pop this in the microwave for a few minutes, and you will have a warm, hearty breakfast to get your day started.

Ingredients:

2 drops liquid Stevia

3 tbsp. hemp hearts

½ tsp. vanilla extract

¼ c coconut milk

½ tsp. turmeric powder

1 tsp. chia seeds

Instructions:

1. Put all ingredients in a jar.
2. Mix well.
3. Put in the refrigerator for a minimum of four hours. Overnight is better.
4. Open and enjoy!

Blueberry Muffins

These delicious muffins are a great make ahead dish that you can grab as you head out the door. These can be eaten warm or at room temperature. Store either in the fridge or freeze for longer storage.

Ingredients:

Cream Together:

½ tsp. vanilla

4 tbsp. softened cream cheese

½ stick softened butter

Dry Ingredients:

¼ c granulated Swerve

1/8 tsp. xanthan gum

Pinch of cinnamon

1 tsp. baking powder

½ c coconut flour

¼ tsp. salt

Wet Ingredients:

¼ c heavy cream

3 large eggs

Add Last:

2 tsp. granulated Swerve

1/3 c fresh blueberries

Instructions:

1. Your oven needs to be set at 350. Place oven rack in lower third of the oven.
2. Line six muffin tins with paper liners.
3. Add the dry ingredients to small bowl and whisk to break apart any lumps.
4. Mix the cream cheese, vanilla, and butter until light and fluffy.
5. Mix one egg and beat until fluffy.

6. Add 1/3 of the dry ingredients and mix well. Make sure you keep the fluffy texture. This needs to be the texture of mousse.
7. Add another egg and beat until completely combined and fluffy.
8. Add half of the remaining ingredients and start beating again.
9. Add the remaining egg, beat until completely incorporated.
10. Use the last of the dry ingredients.
11. Finish this by adding heavy cream and beat until batter is thick but fluffy and light.
12. Fold in blueberries.
13. Spoon batter into muffin liner until about ¾ full.
14. Add any remaining batter to any that might be a little shy.
15. Smooth out tops with a finger.
16. Sprinkle Swerve on the top of each.
17. Put in an oven.
18. Turn up the oven to 400 for five minutes.
19. Turn the oven down to 350 for 25 minutes.
20. Remove from the oven and cool five minutes.
21. Gently remove them from the pan and put on cooling rack.

Zucchini and Bacon Eggs in a Nest

This is a twist on the classic dish eggs in a hole. Since low carb eaters can't have the bread, this recipe substitutes zucchini for the bread and trust me; you don't miss the bread at all.

Ingredients:

Pepper

4 c zucchini noodles

Salt

4 slices bacon

4 eggs

½ c Asiago cheese, grated

Instructions:

1. Cut the bacon in half and then lengthwise into ¼-inch strips.
2. Cook bacon in a heavy sauté pan until desired crispiness.
3. Add zucchini and mix. Add pepper and salt.
4. Flatten out slightly.
5. Make four indentations for the eggs to fit into.
6. Sprinkle with Asiago cheese.
7. Crack one egg into each indentation.
8. Cook about three minutes. Cover. Cook until eggs are done.
9. The bottom should be crispy.
10. Cut into four servings.
11. Serve hot.

Oatmeal

This "oatmeal" is wonderfully satisfying and filling. This will keep you going all day. If you don't like cold oatmeal, pop in the microwave for a couple of minutes.

Ingredients:
3 tbsp. hemp hearts
1 tsp. chia seeds
¼ c heavy whipping cream
1 tbsp. protein powder
Instructions:
1. Put all ingredients in a jar.
2. Mix well.
3. Put in the refrigerator for a minimum of four hours. Overnight is better.
4. Open and enjoy!

Spinach Quiche

Quiche can be eaten for either breakfast or dinner. This is easy to change up flavors you like. If you aren't a fan of spinach, substitute whatever green vegetable you like. This is another great meal to make ahead and portion out into individual portions to grab and go.

Ingredients:

Pepper

1 tbsp. coconut oil

1 package frozen spinach, thawed and drained

1 chopped onion

Salt

3 c shredded cheese

8 eggs, beaten

Instructions:

1. Your oven should be at 350. Oil a 9-inch pie plate with coconut oil.
2. Melt coconut oil in a pan.
3. Mix in onions. Sauté until soft.
4. Add spinach and cook until no longer moist.
5. Let cool slightly.
6. Mix eggs, pepper, salt, and cheese in a bowl.
7. Add spinach and mix well.
8. Pour into pie plate and bake 30 minutes.

Feta and Spinach Omelet

Who doesn't love an omelet? This is a satisfying meal to get you going and keep you full for the rest of the day. If you don't like feta, change the cheese to your favorite. Simple as that.

Ingredients:

Salt

1 clove minced garlic

Pepper

3 c fresh spinach

1 c sliced mushrooms

3 large eggs

2 tbsp. butter or ghee

1/3 c feta cheese, crumbled

Instructions:

1. Melt butter or ghee in a pan.
2. Add garlic, salt, and pepper. Cook until fragrant.
3. Add mushrooms and cook until lightly browned. Mix in the spinach and let cook until wilted.
4. Remove from the heat.
5. Place mixture in a bowl.
6. Wipe out any liquid that remains in the pan.
7. Crack eggs into the bowl.
8. Season with pepper and salt to taste.
9. Mix well.
10. Pour into the hot pan that has been greased with ghee.
11. Use a spatula to bring the egg to the center for about 30 seconds.
12. Tilt the pan to cover it with eggs.

13. Lower the heat and continue to cook. Never rush an omelet. It will get dried out. You want a fluffy, soft omelet.
14. When almost cooked through, add spinach mixture and feta cheese to top.
15. Fold in half and cook another minute to warm center.
16. Slide onto a plate and enjoy.

Maple Walnut Oatmeal

If you enjoy pancakes or waffles, this oatmeal will take you there without all those carbs. This deliciously sweet oatmeal will satisfy any sweet tooth out there. For a warm oatmeal, just pop in the microwave for a few minutes.

Ingredients:

1 tsp. chia seeds

3 tbsp. hemp hearts

3 tbsp. almond milk

1 tbsp. chopped walnuts

½ tsp. cinnamon

½ tbsp. sugar-free maple syrup

Instructions:

1. Put all ingredients in a jar.
2. Mix well.
3. Put in the refrigerator for a minimum of four hours. Overnight is better.
4. Open and enjoy!

Tomato and Cheese Frittata

A slight twist on the classic omelet. This frittata is tasty and filling. If you don't like tomatoes, then change out for mushrooms, spinach, or other favorite vegetables. Leftovers can be cut into individual servings and stored in the refrigerator for a grab and go meal.

Ingredients:

Salt

½ medium sliced onion

Pepper

2/3 c feta, crumbled

2/3 c cherry tomatoes, halved

2 tbsp. chopped herbs of choice

6 large eggs

1 tbsp. ghee or butter

Instructions:

1. Your oven should be at 400 degrees.
2. Melt butter or ghee in a pan.
3. Add onion.
4. Cook until browned
5. Put eggs in a bowl. Season with pepper and salt.
6. Add herbs and mix well.
7. Once onion is soft and slightly browned, add eggs and cook until edges begin to set.
8. Top with cheese and tomatoes.
9. Put under the broiler.
10. Cook about 7 minutes until top is set.
11. Remove and let cool slightly.
12. Serve warm.
13. Store any leftovers in the fridge for five days.

Swiss Chard and Tomato Eggs Benedict

A healthy, low carb version of a timeless classic. If you don't like swiss chard or kale, substitute with spinach, collards, or other leafy green. This is a delicious twist that is easy to make.

Ingredients:

Salt

Large bunch swiss chard

Pepper

2 cloves sliced garlic

4 large poached eggs

4 large thick tomato slices

Blender Hollandaise

1/8 tsp. cayenne pepper

4 oz. salted butter

1 to 3 tsp. lemon juice

3 large egg yolks

Optional Toppings:

Paprika

Chopped chives or scallions

Instructions:

To make Hollandaise:

1. Put egg yolks in the blender.
2. Put the top on but remove the center.
3. Melt butter in a pan until no longer foaming.
4. Turn blender on low and slowly pour in butter.
5. As the sauce begins to emulsify, pour faster.
6. Add lemon juice and pepper.
7. Turn blender on high.
8. Scrape down sides and put the middle back into the lid.
9. Keep sauce in the blender until ready to use.

Swiss Chard or Kale:
1. Wash, remove ribs and cut into 2-inch pieces.
2. Add garlic to hot pan and cook until fragrant.
3. Add kale or swiss chard, cook, until wilted.
4. Add pepper and salt.
5. Once finished, turn off heat and cover.

Poached Eggs:
1. Fill a large frying pan three-quarters of the way full of water, add two teaspoons vinegar and 1 teaspoon salt.
2. Heat until it gets to a slow simmer.
3. Keep temp on medium.
4. Crack each egg gently into the water.
5. Do not let the water boil!
6. Allow to cook two minutes.
7. Turn the eggs over gently and cook until done.
8. Take it out of the pan and drain on a paper towel.

How to Assemble:
1. Place a tomato slice onto a plate.
2. Season with pepper and salt.
3. Divide the greens into four even portions.
4. Place on top of tomatoes.
5. Put poached eggs on top of greens, season with pepper and salt.
6. Drizzle with Hollandaise
7. Garnish as desired.
8. Enjoy.

Double Chocolate Oatmeal

This oatmeal is a must for chocolate lovers. This will satisfy any sweet tooth and keep you feeling full. It will give you the energy to get through your day. If you want a warm oatmeal, pop it in the microwave for a few minutes. Stir and enjoy.

Ingredients:

2 drops liquid stevia

3 tbsp. hemp hearts

1 tsp. chia seeds

1 tbsp. cocoa powder

¼ cup heavy whipping cream

½ tbsp. dark chocolate chips

¼ tsp. salt (add right before eating)

Instructions:

1. Add all ingredients to a jar.
2. Give it a good stir.
3. Put a lid on the jar.
4. Place in the refrigerator for four hours. Overnight is better.
5. Open and enjoy!

All Day Breakfast

This hearty breakfast gives you the energy to get through your entire day. If you love steak and eggs for breakfast, which you can have, this is just a lighter version. The meat will not be missed in this recipe at all.

Ingredients:

Salt

Fresh herbs of choice

Pepper

1 large egg

1 tbsp. butter or ghee

3 slices bacon

½ avocado

2 large Portobello mushrooms

Instructions:

1. Melt one-half tablespoon butter or ghee in a pan.
2. Add mushrooms, sprinkle with pepper and salt and cook until tender.
3. Wipe out any water that remains in a pan.
4. Fry bacon until desired consistency.
5. Drain grease.
6. Melt rest of butter or ghee.
7. Fry eggs to your liking.
8. Plate everything and enjoy.

Brie and Bacon Frittata

Frittatas are a wonderfully filling and satisfying breakfast dish. If you don't like brie, substitute your favorite cheese. This can be cut into portions and stored in the refrigerator for another grab and go dish.

Ingredients:

4 oz. thinly sliced brie

8 slices bacon

½ tsp. pepper

8 large eggs

½ tsp. salt

½ c whipping cream

2 cloves minced garlic

Instructions:

1. Cook bacon until as crisp as you like it.
2. Drain on a paper towel.
3. Keep the bacon grease in the skillet.
4. Take skillet off of the heat.
5. In a large bowl, mix eggs, pepper, salt, garlic, cream and about 2/3 of crumbled bacon.
6. Put the skillet back on heat and swirl grease to coat bottom and sides.
7. Put eggs in the skillet and cook. Do not touch!!
8. Wait until edges are set, and center is still loose.
9. This will take about ten minutes.
10. Heat the broiler.
11. Put slices of brie on top of the frittata.
12. Sprinkle with the rest of bacon.
13. Broil until puffy and golden. Watch closely, so it doesn't burn.
14. Remove from the oven and allow to cool for a few minutes.
15. Serve and enjoy!

Almond Joy Oatmeal

My favorite candy bar of all times has to be Almond Joys. This oatmeal takes me back to my childhood and simpler days. This is a hearty, satisfying oatmeal that will give you the energy to tackle your day. To have a warm oatmeal for chilly mornings, just pop in the microwave for a few minutes. If you don't like stevia any sweetener of choice will do.

Ingredients:

1 drop liquid stevia

3 tbsp. hemp hearts

¼ c coconut milk

½ tbsp. chopped almonds

½ tbsp. shredded coconut

½ tbsp. chocolate chips

Instructions:

1. Put all ingredients in a pint jar.
2. Stir to combine.
3. Place in the refrigerator for four hours. Overnight is better.
4. Open and enjoy!

Cream Cheese and Salmon Mug Muffin

This quick and easy recipe just takes a few ingredients and a mug. Mug cakes, muffins, etc. are all the rage these days. And it is easy to understand why. Just mix everything and pop in the microwave. Easy peasy.

Ingredients:

Salt

2 tbsp. water

2 tbsp. chopped chives or scallions

2 tbsp. cream

¼ c almond flour

1 large egg

¼ c flax meal

¼ tsp. baking soda

2 oz. smoked salmon, thinly sliced

Top with 2 dollops of sour cream

Instructions:

1. Put almond flour, flax meal, and baking soda in a microwave safe mug.
2. Put egg, water, and cream into small bowl.
3. Mix well with a fork.
4. Add smoked salmon and combine well.
5. Pour into a mug and stir well to combine all ingredients.
6. Microwave on high 60 to 90 seconds.
7. Once done, top with sour cream and enjoy.

Sausage and Kale Hash

If you love hash, this is a great alternative. This recipe is versatile. So feel free to substitute whatever greens you like. If you aren't a fan of poached eggs, just fry them to your liking.

Ingredients:

Salt

7 oz. kale

Pepper

1 tsp. Dijon mustard

2 c cauliflower rice

2 cloves garlic, minced

1 tbsp. lemon juice

3 tbsp. lard or ghee

5 oz. sausage

Toppings:

4 poached eggs

Instructions:

1. Rice the cauliflower in a food processor.
2. Cut ribs out of kale and chop.
3. Melt ghee in the skillet.
4. Cook sausage until thoroughly cooked. Transfer to the bowl.
5. Add remaining ghee to the pan.
6. Put in the garlic and cook until fragrant.
7. Add cauliflower rice and cook for five minutes. Stir to keep from burning.
8. Add kale, Dijon, lemon juice, cook two minutes more and continue to stir.
9. Season with pepper and salt.
10. Mix to combine.
11. Once done, add sausage back into the pan and mix well.
12. Remove from the heat.
13. Place eggs on top.

Pumpkin Pie Oatmeal

If you love pumpkin spice everything, then you are going to fall in love with this recipe. This hearty oatmeal is flavored with the flavors of fall and Thanksgiving. Just pop in the microwave for a bit to have a warm and delicious breakfast.

Ingredients:

1 tbsp. pumpkin puree

3 tbsp. hemp hearts

3 tbsp. almond milk

½ tsp. pumpkin pie spice

2 drops liquid stevia

1 tsp. chia seeds

Instructions:

1. Place everything in a pint jar.
2. Stir to combine.
3. Put in the refrigerator for a minimum of four hours. Overnight is better.
4. Open and enjoy!

Shamrock Eggs

This is a great St. Patrick's Day breakfast. It could even be used to celebrate Dr. Seuss's birthday. You can read Green Eggs and Ham to your child while they eat. It's an easy way to get them to eat their vegetables, too.

Ingredients:

Salt

½ diced red onion

Pepper

2 large green bell pepper rings

1 tbsp. ghee

1 c baby spinach

¼ c sliced bacon

2 large eggs

Instructions:

1. Remove seeds and ribs from bell pepper.
2. Slice into 1-inch slices.
3. Pick two slices from the center of the bell pepper.
4. Eat the rest with breakfast or use in a salad.
5. Place ½ tablespoon of ghee in a pan and cook the bell pepper rings for three minutes.
6. Break an egg into each ring.
7. Sprinkle with pepper and salt.
8. Cook eggs to your liking.
9. In different pan, melt remaining ghee
10. Add onion.
11. Cook until tender.
12. Add bacon and cook until desired consistency.
13. Add spinach and salt.
14. Cook for a few more minutes.
15. Plate everything and enjoy.

Pizza Muffin

This recipe will take care of your pizza cravings. These can be made in advance and stored in the fridge. Take one out of the fridge and eat it at room temperature or pop in the microwave for a few seconds.

Ingredients:

2-oz pepperoni

½ tsp. baking soda

½ tsp. sea salt

4 eggs

½ c Parmesan

¼ c tomato sauce

½ c cheddar cheese

1 ½ c almond flour

Instructions:

1. Your oven should be at 350.
2. Combine the salt, flour, and baking soda in a food processor.
3. Add the eggs, pepperoni, and both kinds of cheese.
4. Pulse until well combined.
5. Place liners in a muffin tin.
6. Add four tablespoons of batter into every cup.
7. Continue until all batter is used.
8. Bake for 25 minutes.
9. Once done, top with a teaspoon of sauce, extra cheese, and pepperoni.
10. Cook for another 15 minutes.

Crepes

This is a light version of the classic crepe. These can be filled with your favorite low carb filling. A good smear of cream cheese and some strawberries down the center is absolutely delicious.

Ingredients:

4 eggs

1 tbsp. coconut oil

½ c water

2 tbsp. coconut oil, for cooking

2 tbsp. coconut flour

Instructions:

1. Mix the eggs and flour in a food processor.
2. Pulse in a tablespoon of oil and water.
3. Heat some oil in an 8-inch pan.
4. Place four tablespoons of the batter in the pan and rotate so that it covers the bottom.
5. When bubbles form, flip, and cook the other side until done.
6. Place crepe on a plate.
7. Continue with rest of batter.

Italian Omelet

If you love everything flavored Italian, you are going to love this delicious, hearty omelet. If you aren't a fan of Sopressata, substitute your favorite Italian meats and cheeses.

Ingredients:

Salt

1 tbsp. water

Pepper

2 eggs

2 oz. mozzarella

1 tbsp. butter

5 slices ripe tomato

6 basil leaves

3 slices Sopressata

Instructions:

1. Whisk eggs and water together.
2. Melt butter in nonstick pan.
3. Put eggs in a pan and cook 30 seconds.
4. Put meat onto one-half of the egg.
5. Add basil, tomato, and cheese.
6. Season with pepper and salt.
7. Cook an additional two minutes until egg is firm and will fold over ingredients.
8. Gently fold in half.
9. Cover and cook on low about two minutes more.
10. Slide omelet onto a plate and enjoy.

Porridge

This cousin of oatmeal is a creamier alternative that is flavored with cinnamon and chia seeds. Adding raisins, sunflower seeds, and coconut to the top add some crunch and sweetness.

Ingredients:

1 tbsp. flax seed

1 tsp. cinnamon

1 tbsp. pumpkin seeds

1 c boiling water

1 tbsp. chia seeds

¼ c walnuts

¼ tsp. sea salt

2 tbsp. unsweetened coconut

Instructions:

1. Put all dry ingredients in a food processor and pulse until it is finely ground.
2. Pour in water and blend; slowly moving from low to high, until it gets smooth and creamy.
3. Place in a bowl and top with extra coconut, sunflower seeds, and raisins.

Chili Cheese Muffins

If spicy foods are what you love, then these spicy little tidbits are for you. Start your day with these spicy muffins and enjoy the rest of your day. These can also be a spicy sidekick to a nice bowl of chili to finish your day.

Ingredients:

½ tsp. sea salt

2 c packed cheddar cheese

½ tsp. baking soda

1 ¼ c almond flour

2 tbsp. red pepper flakes

3 eggs

Instructions:

1. Your oven should be at 350.
2. Add the salt, flour, and baking soda to a food processor.
3. Add eggs and pulse until they are mixed well.
4. Now add cheese and a tablespoon of the pepper flakes.
5. Pulse again until completely combined.
6. Place paper cups in a muffin tin and put four tablespoons of the batter into each.
7. Sprinkle with the rest of the pepper flakes.
8. Cook for 25 to 30 minutes.

Green Eggs

This is a great breakfast to serve for Dr. Seuss's birthday or on St. Patrick's Day. The name sounds unappealing, but these are packed with flavor and fiber to get your day going. These will keep you full to get those errands done and then some.

Ingredients:

Oil

4 eggs

Sea salt

4 large kale leaves

Instructions:

1. Add salt, eggs, and kale to a food processor.
2. Blend until well combined.
3. Warm oil in a skillet.
4. Pour in eggs and cook until done.

Sides

Cauliflower Fritters

These fritters make a great side to any meal or can be eaten alone as a snack. This process might seem daunting, but these come together easily and quickly for a delicious and hearty treat.

Ingredients:

1 ½ tsp. lemon pepper

1 lb. cauliflower

3 large eggs

1 tsp. salt

3 oz. chopped onion

½ c almond flour

½ tsp. baking powder

½ c Parmesan cheese, grated

Instructions:

1. Rice cauliflower in food processor.
2. Place in a bowl, sprinkle with salt.
3. Let sit for 10 minutes.
4. Place chopped onions in a bowl.
5. Squeeze all the water out of cauliflower and put it with the onion.
6. Add almond flour, baking powder, seasonings, and cheese.
7. Combine.
8. Add three eggs and mix again.

Skillet Method:

1. Melt one tablespoon oil in frying pan.
2. Put four tablespoons batter into hot skillet.
3. Pat down with the spatula to make a pancake.
4. Cook about three minutes on each side.

5. Don't flip until bottoms are well browned.
6. Drain on paper towels.

Oven Method:

1. Your oven should be at 400.
2. Place foil on two baking sheets.
3. Put four tablespoons batter at a time on the baking sheet.
4. Shape into either circles or rectangles.
5. Bake about 12 minutes.
6. Gently, turn them over and bake for 12 more minutes.
7. Store any leftovers in the fridge.
8. Reheat in a dry skillet to make them crispy again.

Cauliflower Mac and Cheese

If you are a mac and cheese lover, this will become your new favorite. You do not miss the pasta in this tasty dish. Feel free to change up the cheese to suit you. No carbs and plenty of healthy fats.

Ingredients:

Ghee

½ tsp. pepper

1/8 tsp. garlic powder

1 ½ cups shredded cheddar cheese

1 cauliflower, cut into florets

1 ½ tsp. Dijon mustard

½ cup cottage cheese

1 tsp. salt

½ to ¾ cup kefir

Instructions:

1. Your oven should be at 375. Grease 8X8 pan with ghee.
2. Bring a pot of salted water to a boil.
3. Put cauliflower in and cook until tender.
4. Drain and let dry while you fix the cheese sauce.
5. Place in the prepared pan.
6. In a saucepan mix kefir, cottage cheese, and mustard until smooth.
7. Stir in garlic powder, pepper, salt, and cheese until cheese begins to melt.
8. Pour over cauliflower and stir to coat.
9. Top with more cheese.
10. Bake until bubbly and slightly browned.

Kale Slaw

This is a simple recipe with only three ingredients. The hardest part is prepping the vegetables. It is a perfect side to a good saucy barbecue and big side of ribs. Kale gives this recipe a new taste on an old classic.

Ingredients:

¼ cup almonds, chopped

4 carrots

2 heads kale

Instructions:

1. Remove the ribs from the kale
2. Slice into strips.
3. Julienne the carrots.
4. Toss everything together.
5. Add your favorite coleslaw dressing.
6. Mix well and enjoy.

Cheesy Risotto

For those of you who love creamy, cheesy risotto but hate standing over the stove until it's done, this is a quick and tasty way to have it without the carbs.

Ingredients:

Salt

4 tbsp. chopped chives or scallions

1 c shredded cheddar cheese

1 c grated Parmesan cheese

½ c butter or ghee

1 tsp. Dijon mustard

1 finely chopped small white onion

6 c cauliflower rice

1 c chicken or vegetable stock

Instructions:

1. Rice the cauliflower by processing it in a food processor until it resembles rice.
2. Do not cook the cauliflower.
3. Melt butter in large pan.
4. Add the chopped onion and cook until soft.
5. Mix in the cauliflower rice and mix.
6. Cook a few minutes and pour in the stock.
7. Cook five minutes until the cauliflower rice is tender crisp.
8. Add mustard, mix well and remove from the heat.
9. Set some Parmesan and chives to the side for garnish.
10. Add the rest to the pan.
11. Mix well.
12. Taste and add more salt if needed.
13. Place in bowls and top with Parmesan and chives.
14. Serve hot!

Cheesy Garlic Creamed Spinach

Most people aren't a fan of creamed spinach. Try this recipe, and it will change your mind. This is a delicious cheesy version of the old lunchroom classic. The goat cheese gives it a wonderful tanginess that excites your taste buds.

Ingredients:

¼ c goat cheese

1 c heavy cream

¼ c grated Parmesan cheese

Pepper

Salt

2 lbs. fresh spinach

3 tbsp. butter

¼ c shredded mozzarella cheese

4 cloves minced garlic

Instructions:

1. Melt butter in sauté pan.
2. Add garlic and cook until fragrant.
3. Mix in spinach.
4. Season with pepper and salt.
5. Cook until wilted.
6. Remove and drain.
7. Squeeze out all moisture.
8. In the same pan, add heavy cream, goat cheese, mozzarella, and Parmesan.
9. Lower the heat and simmer the sauce until thick.
10. Add spinach to the pan and toss to coat.

Spicy Slaw

If you love your barbecue spicy, then this is the perfect side for you. This is not a mayonnaise based slaw. This one is dressed with a vinaigrette that gives a whole new spin on slaw.

Ingredients:

2 limes, juiced

Sea salt

7 drops stevia

½ purple cabbage, shredded

1 tsp. ginger, minced

1 minced jalapeno

2 tbsp. olive oil

1 grated carrot

Bunch Cilantro, chopped

Instructions:

1. Put the cabbage, carrot, Cilantro, and jalapeno in a large bowl.
2. Mix to combine.
3. Whisk together olive oil, ginger, stevia, salt, and lime juice.
4. Pour over the vegetables.
5. Toss well to coat.

No-Potato Salad

This is a perfect substitution for the classic picnic side. I love my potato salad, and with this recipe, I can trick my taste buds into thinking they are chowing down on some good old homemade potato salad.

Ingredients:

½ tsp. sea salt

2 diced stalks of celery

1 tbsp. Dijon

1 small chopped onion

2 tbsp. mayonnaise

1 head cauliflower

2 hard-boiled eggs, diced

1 tbsp. parsley, chopped

Instructions:

1. Break cauliflower into florets.
2. Steam or cook until tender.
3. If you are boiling cauliflower, drain completely.
4. Let sit to finish draining.
5. Cool the cauliflower slightly.
6. Mix in the remaining ingredients.

Asparagus Basil Salad

My family was never a big fan of asparagus until I made this gem. This salad is so flavorful; your family will be begging for it again and again.

Ingredients:

½ tsp. pepper

1 lb. asparagus, trimmed and diced

1 c basil leaves, sliced

1 avocado, cubed

½ tsp. sea salt

2 tsp. Dijon

¼ c olive oil

1 c grape tomatoes, halved

2 tsp. lemon juice

Instructions:

1. Steam the asparagus until tender.
2. Toss everything together.
3. Season with pepper and salt.
4. Give it a taste test and season again if needed.

Buttery Broccoli

This simple side is a quick and easy complement to any entrée. With just four ingredients this is ready to be put on the table in no time.

Ingredients:

Salt

1 large head broccoli, cut up including stalk

Pepper

¼ c butter, cut into cubes

Instructions:

1. Set butter out on the counter to soften while cooking broccoli.

2. Steam or cook broccoli in salted water.

3. If steaming, sprinkle with salt before placing in the steamer.

4. Cook until tender.

5. Drain.

6. Add broccoli and butter to the bowl and toss to coat.

7. Add some salt and pepper to taste.

8. Serve and enjoy!

Green Bean Tapenade

If you have never tried tapenade on green beans, you are in for a treat. This enhances the flavor of the green beans to a level you will want them every day. This quick and easy side will go with any entrée you care to make.

Ingredients:

Pepper

1 ½ lb. green beans, remove ends

½ cup black olive tapenade

Salt

Instructions:

1. Allow a medium pot of water to come to a boil.
2. Place the green beans and boil about 5 minutes.
3. Once beans are done, strain and allow to dry.
4. Toss with tapenade until well coated.
5. Season with pepper and salt.
6. Serve and enjoy!

Appetizers
Mushroom Soup

You will never use canned cream of mushroom soup again. This recipe is quick and tasty. You could also thicken it and use it as a gravy over Salisbury steak. If you don't like shiitake mushrooms, use what you like.

Ingredients:

½ tsp. sea salt

1 lb. shiitake mushrooms, chopped

2 tbsp. olive oil

1 chopped medium onion

8 c chicken stock

Instructions:

1. Warm a stock pot.
2. Add oil.
3. Cook onions until browned.
4. Add mushrooms and cook until soft.
5. Put in the stock and let boil.
6. Reduce heat to a simmer.
7. Simmer ten minutes.
8. In batches, blend in a blender until everything is smooth.
9. You can also use an immersion blender if you have one.

Avocado Deviled Eggs

Who doesn't love deviled eggs? These are the greatest, tastiest morsels to have at any gathering or at any time really. These are great to use as a quick energy booster as well. Loaded with healthy fats that will give you the energy to finish your day.

Ingredients:

2 tbsp. chopped chives or scallions

¼ c mayonnaise

½ large avocado

1 tbsp. lemon juice

3 large cooked eggs

Pepper

Salt

Instructions:

1. Cook the eggs.
2. Gently place eggs in a saucepan.
3. Cover with water.
4. Add salt, and allow to come to a boil.
5. Boil 10 minutes.
6. When done, remove from the heat and put in cold water.
7. Peel when they have chilled.
8. Run a sharp knife around the outside of the avocado to cut it in half.
9. Carefully remove the pit and peel.
10. Slice the eggs in half and carefully remove the yolk.
11. Put the yolks in the bowl of a food processor.
12. Add the avocado to the food processor along with the egg yolks, pepper, salt, lemon juice, and mayonnaise.

13. Process until completely smooth.
14. You could mash everything together with a fork until creamy.
15. Fill the whites with yolk and avocado mixture to make the deviled eggs.
16. Add the chopped chives to the top.
17. Place in an airtight container in the refrigerator to prevent browning for up to five days.
18. Any leftover filling tastes great on top of cucumber slices.

Prosciutto Wrapped Mozzarella

Roommate calls and says they're bringing home the boss? What do you do? Go grab some mozzarella balls, basil leaves, and prosciutto and make this quick and easy appetizer to satisfy the hungriest of the hungry.

Ingredients:

Pepper

Salt

18 fresh basil leaves

6 thin slices prosciutto

18 small mozzarella

Instructions:

1. Slice prosciutto into 1-inch pieces.
2. Lay the slices out.
3. Place a basil leaf on each strip.
4. Place a mozzarella ball on each basil leaf.
5. Sprinkle with pepper and salt.
6. Roll up and serve.

Nachos

If your favorite game day food is nachos, this recipe will make your day. This is your new go to recipe for nachos. Carb free and loaded with healthy fats and proteins our bodies need.

Ingredients:

For Tortilla Chips:

Salt

1 ¾ c shredded mozzarella

Pinch chili powder

¾ c almond flour

1 tsp. coriander powder

1 egg

1 tsp. cumin powder

2 tbsp. cream cheese

For Meat Sauce:

1 tbsp. tomato paste

1 diced red onion

½ tsp. chili powder

1lb ground beef

14 oz. diced tomatoes

Optional Toppings:

Jalapenos

Guacamole

Sour cream

Salsa

Shredded cheese

Instructions:

Meat Sauce:

1. Warm oil in a pan.
2. Add onion cook until softened.
3. Add meat, spices, tomato paste, and diced tomatoes.

4. Mix well.
5. Simmer about 15 minutes.

Tortilla Chips:
1. Your oven needs to be at 425.
2. While the meat is cooking, put the almond flour and shredded cheese in a microwaveable bowl.
3. Add cream cheese to the bowl.
4. Microwave for one minute.
5. Stir well.
6. Microwave for another 30 seconds.
7. Take out and stir again.
8. Add spices, salt, and egg.
9. Mix well.
10. Place the mixture between two sheets of parchment paper and roll thin.
11. Remove the top sheet of parchment paper.
12. Place the bottom sheet of parchment paper onto a baking sheet.
13. Bake 15 minutes until brown.
14. Take out of the oven.
15. Carefully flip over onto another piece of parchment and brown this side.
16. Once both sides are browned, take out of the oven and cut into triangles.
17. Bake the triangles another five minutes.

Put it Together:
1. Put chips on a plate.
2. Put some meat mixture on top.
3. Add some shredded cheese.
4. Add the toppings of choice.
5. Serve with a side salad and enjoy!

Salmon Bites

If you love ordering crab cakes as an appetizer, these are a great second. You can add any other spices you would like or just keep it simple with the dill. This recipe is great for serving at any gathering.

Ingredients:

2 oz. cream cheese

½ tsp. salt

1 tsp. dried dill

½ c shredded cheese

2 oz. smoked salmon, sliced

6 eggs

Instructions:

1. Your oven should be set at 350.
2. Grease a mini muffin tin.
3. Whisk eggs, milk, and salt together.
4. Add dill, chopped cream cheese, salmon, and shredded cheese.
5. Pour in the greased mini muffin a pan.
6. Allow them to cook at 350 for about 15 minutes.
7. Let cool before removing from the pan.

Chive and Garlic Sunflower Seed Cheese

Brie is a fancy addition to any cheese platter. This tastes just as good, and it is full of healthy fats which are a big score. So, the next time you need to impress a client or boss, bring out this on a platter, and you have just earned plenty of brownie points.

Ingredients:

½ c chives, rough chopped

6 tbsp. extra virgin olive oil

½ c lemon juice

2 c raw sunflower seeds

2 tsp. salt

2 cloves garlic

Instructions:

1. Put sunflower seeds and a teaspoon of salt in water and soak overnight.
2. Drain and rinse.
3. Put in food processor and process smooth.
4. Add remaining ingredients and blend until combined and smooth.
5. Enjoy!

**You can bake this like you would brie. Heat oven to 200. Spread on a lined baking sheet, or shape into a circle that is around three-fourths of an inch thick. Bake for 45 minutes. The top and sides will be firm, but the inside will be soft and spreadable.

Bread

This isn't an appetizer, but I felt like it was important to add it in since bread is so often missed by keto dieters. Once sliced, you can use as toast or a sandwich. You can use this just like normal bread.

Ingredients:

Pinch salt

¼ tsp. cream of tartar

1 ½ c almond flour

3 tsp. baking powder

6 large eggs, separated

4 tbsp. melted butter

Instructions:

1. Your oven needs to be at 375.
2. Separate the egg yolks from the whites.
3. Put egg whites in a bowl and add cream of tartar.
4. Beat with hand mixer until soft peaks have formed.
5. Put egg yolks, a third of the egg whites, salt, baking powder, almond flour, and melted butter in a food processor.
6. Process until just combined.
7. It will be lumpy and thick until the egg whites are added.
8. Add the rest of the egg whites and pulse until combined well.
9. Make sure not to overmix.
10. The egg whites will give the bread volume.
11. Put into a buttered loaf pan.
12. Bake for 30 minutes.
13. Check with toothpick for doneness.
14. One loaf will make 20 slices.
15. Enjoy!

Broccoli Soup

This is a good way to get your children to eat vegetables. It is also an elegant way to begin a dinner party. You won't taste the broccoli with the other flavors in this soup.

Ingredients:

½ tsp. sea salt

2 tbsp. olive oil

1 ½ lb. broccoli

8 c water

1 medium chopped onion, chopped

Instructions:

1. Sauté onions until soft.
2. Add broccoli and cook five minutes.
3. Add water and salt and cook another 15 minutes.
4. Put in a blender and puree until smooth.
5. You can also use an immersion blender.

Buffalo Chicken Salad Sandwiches

Everyone loves buffalo chicken wings. These sandwiches are just the thing without the bones. You could also substitute blue cheese dressing if you prefer.

Ingredients:

For Quick Bun:

1 tsp. baking powder

2 tbsp. butter

4 eggs, beaten

2 ½ tbsp. coconut flour, sifted

3 ½ tbsp. heavy cream

2 ½ tbsp. golden flax meal

For Chicken Salad:

4 tbsp. ranch dressing

2 c cooked shredded chicken

3 tbsp. mayonnaise

1/3 c hot sauce

2 tbsp. minced celery

3 tbsp. butter

¼ tsp. salt

¼ tsp. celery seed

¼ tsp. garlic powder

Instructions:

1. Your oven needs to set on 400.
2. Grease 4 glass ramekins.
3. In a bowl, put all the bun ingredients and stir vigorously.
4. Scrape down the sides and break up lumps.
5. Divide the batter equally into each ramekin.
6. Bake about 15 minutes until center is done.
7. Remove from the oven and cool completely.

8. Cut the buns in half sandwich style.
9. If you would like, you can toast these.
10. In a saucepan add butter, salt, garlic powder, celery seed, and hot sauce.
11. Stir continuously until melted and combined.
12. Put in the cooked chicken and celery and stir.
13. Remove from the heat.
14. Add mayonnaise and mix to combine.

To make the sandwiches

1. Put one half cup chicken mixture on each bun.
2. Add ranch dressing to the top.
3. Serve and enjoy.

Baked Salami and Cheese

Here is another quick and easy appetizer for game day. This is tasty and looks fancy for any buffet table.

Ingredients:

¼ c chopped parsley

4 oz. cream cheese, flavored if you want

7 oz. dried salami

Instructions:

1. Your oven should be at 325.
2. Line baking sheet with aluminum foil.
3. Cut the salami into 30 slices that are one-quarter of an inch thick.
4. Place on baking sheet.
5. Do not overlap the pieces.
6. Bake 15 minutes.
7. Put on paper towels and let cool.
8. Top each salami piece with some cream cheese and parsley.

Pepper Nachos

This is a great way to enjoy the flavors of nachos without all the carbs. Baking the mini peppers makes them sweet and flavorful. The taco meat on them takes nachos to a whole other level. You will not miss the chips with this recipe.

Ingredients:

1 tbsp. chili powder

½ tsp. salt

½ c chopped tomato

1 ½ c shredded Cheddar cheese

½ tsp. oregano

1 lb. mini pepper, seeded and halved

1 lb. ground beef

1 tsp. cumin

¼ tsp. red pepper flakes

1 tsp. garlic powder

½ tsp. pepper

1 tsp. paprika

Additional toppings:

Olives

Avocado

Sour cream

Jalapeno, chopped

Instructions:

1. Add all spices to the bowl. Mix well to combine.
2. Cook ground beef until no longer pink.
3. Break up any lumps.
4. Drain.
5. Add mixed spices and ½ cup water.
6. Cook until water is absorbed.

7. Take off heat.
8. Your oven should be at 400.
9. Put foil on a large baking sheet.
10. Put mini peppers in a single layer, cut side up.
11. Add ground beef mixture to peppers.
12. Top with shredded cheese.
13. Bake until cheese is melted.
14. Take out of the oven and top with desired toppings.
15. Serve and enjoy.

Green Soup

Here is another soup that is creamy and healthy. A great way to get your vegetables without really tasting them. If you don't like collards, switch it out for a different green.

Ingredients:

1 tbsp. lemon juice

2 tbsp. olive oil

2 tbsp. ginger, minced

1 medium chopped onion

Bunch Collards

8 c chicken stock

2 leeks, sliced

1 tsp. sea salt

Instructions:

1. Warm oil in large pot.
2. Cook onions until soft.
3. Add leeks and cook ten minutes.
4. Add the ginger and cook until fragrant.
5. Add collards and cook until wilted.
6. Add stock and cook another ten minutes.
7. Using an immersion blender, blend until the soup is smooth.
8. Place back in the pot, heat thoroughly, and mix in the lemon juice.

Smoothies

Red Velvet Smoothie

This smoothie will replace your urge for cake since this smoothie tastes just like a slice of red velvet cake. This will soon become your favorite drink first thing in the mornings.

Ingredients:

3 tbsp. cocoa powder

½ small beet

2 tbsp. sweetener

½ avocado

2 c coconut milk

¼ tsp. vanilla

2 c ice

Instructions:

1. Run a knife around the outside of the avocado to open.
2. Carefully remove the pit.
3. Add everything to the blender.
4. Blend until creamy and smooth.
5. Taste and add more sweetener if needed.
6. If you don't have a powerful blender, boil the beet first.
7. If you don't want red hands, wear gloves when peeling and handling the beet.

Chocolate Covered Strawberry Smoothie

Don't worry about not getting chocolates for special occasions. You don't need them with this recipe. This smoothie is so rich and creamy and packed full of protein to get you through your day

Ingredients:

7 ice cubes

2 scoops protein powder

2 c coconut milk

1 c strawberries

¼ c cocoa powder

Instructions:

1. Wash and hull the strawberries.
2. Put the cocoa, protein powder, strawberries, and milk into the blender.
3. Once it has become smooth, add one ice cube.
4. Blend until smooth and creamy.
5. Once the smoothie is the consistency you like, stop adding ice.
6. Pour into a glass and enjoy.

Power Smoothie

With all the protein packed ingredients in this smoothie, you are going to have enough energy to get you through the day and then some.

Ingredients:

3 ice cubes

1 c frozen strawberries

1 tbsp. chia seeds, ground

½ c Kevita probiotic drink, coconut

1 scoop protein powder

1 tbsp. almond butter

5 drops vanilla stevia

Instructions:

1. Add all ingredients to a blender.
2. Blend until everything is creamy and smooth.

Strawberry Rhubarb Smoothie

This smoothie brings me back to my childhood days when my mom would buy and strawberry and rhubarb pie. There is nothing quite as refreshing as this combination on a hot day.

Ingredients:

2 tbsp. coconut milk

3 to 6 drops liquid stevia

3 strawberries

1 tsp. fresh ginger

1 rhubarb stalk, diced

½ c almond milk

2 tbsp. almond butter

1 egg

½ tsp. vanilla

3 to 4 cubes of ice

Instructions:

1. Add vanilla, egg, almond butter, diced rhubarb, strawberries, stevia, coconut milk, almond milk, and ginger to a blender.
2. Blend until smooth.
3. Add ice one cube at a time until you have it as thick as you want it.

Peanut Butter Protein Smoothie

If you love peanut butter, you are going to fall madly in love with this smoothie. Packed full of protein and good fats, it will give you the boost you need to accomplish everything on your to do list.

Ingredients:

1 tbsp. peanut butter

2 drops Stevia

½ cup cottage cheese

1 c ice

½ cup almond milk

Instructions:

1. Add everything except the ice to your blender.
2. Blend until creamy.
3. Add ice a few cubes at a time until as thick as you want it.

Pumpkin Keto Smoothie

If you love everything pumpkin flavored, then you are going to love this smoothie. This smoothie tastes like fall. It has added protein to give you that boost to get through the holidays.

Ingredients:

1 tbsp. MCT oil

½ c coconut milk

¼ c pumpkin puree

¼ c whey protein

1 tsp. erythritol

½ tsp. pumpkin pie spice

¼ c almond milk

Instructions:

1. Add all ingredients to a blender.
2. Blend until everything is incorporated and it's nice a creamy.

Strawberry Smoothie

This is the closest drink to having a strawberry milkshake. You don't miss the carbs or calories in this sweet, refreshing smoothie.

Ingredients:

¼ c coconut milk

½ c strawberries

½ tsp. vanilla

1 tbsp. MCT or coconut oil

¾ c almond milk

Instructions:

1. Wash and hull the strawberries.
2. Add to blender.
3. Add milk and blend smooth.
4. Add the remaining ingredients and pulse a few more times.

Shamrock Shake

This is the best healthy mint shake you will ever have. You definitely aren't going to miss the calories in this baby. This would be great for those hot summer days when you need a refreshing boost. Of course, this needs to be served on St. Patrick's Day.

Ingredients:

½ avocado

1 c ice

½ tsp. salt

2 tbsp. cream cheese

¾ c coconut milk

1 tsp. stevia

¼ tsp. mint extract

¼ c protein powder

Instructions:

1. Run a knife around avocado and twist to open.
2. Carefully remove pit.
3. Peel and place in the blender.
4. Add remaining ingredients and blend until creamy and delicious.

Faux Frosty

If you love getting a frosty with your meal, this one is great because it doesn't have all the extra calories and sugar. You get an extra boost from the protein powder to help you with your daily chores.

Ingredients:

¾ c almond milk

1 scoop vanilla protein powder

2 tbsp. cocoa powder

¼ tsp. guar gum

Choice of sweetener

15 ice cubes

Instructions:

1. Add all the ingredients except ice into a blender.
2. Blend until creamy and smooth.
3. Add ice a few cubes at a time until it is as thick as you want.

Chocolate Cherry Smoothie

If your favorite holiday treat is chocolate covered cherries, then this is the drink for you. You don't miss any of the flavors with this smoothie. It is packed full of healthy proteins that will help you do your daily activities.

Ingredients:

½ c cherries

1/3 c hemp hearts

1 scoop protein powder

¼ c cocoa powder

1 c ice

½ tsp. chocolate stevia

1 c coconut milk

Instructions:

1. If your cherries haven't been pitted, do so before placing them in the blender.
2. Add all other ingredients except ice.
3. Blend smooth.
4. Add ice until you have the thickness you want.

Coconut Mocha Frappe

You won't go back to your favorite coffee shop after one taste of this yummy frappe. If you love coffee flavor, this will send you to the moon and back.

Ingredients:

1/3 c ice

2 tsp. instant coffee

1 drop coconut extract

1 packet stevia

½ tsp. cocoa powder

2 c coconut milk

Instructions:

1. Add all ingredients except ice to a blender.
2. Blend until everything is incorporated.
3. Add ice a few cubes at a time until creamy and thick.

Peppermint Hot Chocolate Smoothie

If you are like me, you love putting a candy cane in your hot chocolate while sitting around on cold winter nights. This smoothie takes you there, but you don't have to wait for the holidays. You can have this any day of the year.

Ingredients:

1 ½ c almond milk

½ tsp. peppermint extract

2 c ice

½ tsp. protein powder, chocolate

3 oz. dark chocolate, chopped

1 tsp. peppermint stevia

Instructions:

1. Put everything in a blender except ice.
2. Blend until well combined.
3. Add ice a few cubes at a time until thick and creamy.

Cake Batter Smoothie

You don't need a slice of cake with this smoothie. This is rich, creamy, and delicious. A tasty way to start your day or as a midday pick me up.

Ingredients:

½ c cottage cheese

½ tsp. vanilla

½ tsp. xanthan gum

3 to 5 packets stevia

1 scoop protein powder

1 c water

10 ice cubes

3 to 5 drops almond extract

Instructions:

1. When putting ingredients in the blender, start with the least amount of almond extract and stevia.
2. Don't add ice yet.
3. Blend until combined.
4. Taste and adjust almond extract and sweetener as needed.
5. Add ice a few cubes at a time until thick and creamy.

Main Dishes

Chili Turkey Burgers

This is a healthy version of traditional burgers. You won't miss anything with these burgers. Your family will not know they aren't made with beef unless you tell them.

Ingredients:

1 tsp. sea salt

1 tsp. chili powder

½ c onion, chopped

8 oz. diced green chilies

2 tsp. cumin

1 lb. ground turkey

1 c Cilantro, chopped

Instructions:

1. Put all ingredients into a large bowl.
2. Mix all well by hand and shape into eight patties.
3. Grill or fry until done.
4. Add favorite burger toppings and enjoy.

Chicken Parmesan

This is a delicious twist on an old classic. Serve with some zucchini noodles to make a complete meal. Bake a loaf of keto bread to round it out with some garlic bread.

Ingredients:

16 oz. mozzarella

4 chicken breasts

6 sliced garlic cloves

2 c almond flour

1 tsp. herbs de Provence

2 eggs, beaten

2 c water

6 tbsp. butter

14 oz. tomato paste

Instructions:

1. Heat oven to 400.
2. Slice chicken into cutlets that are fairly thin.
3. Dip each cutlet in the egg and then coat with flour.
4. Melt the butter in an oven proof skillet.
5. Cook the chicken until golden.
6. Remove from the pan.
7. Add the garlic, herbs, water, and tomato paste together to the pan.
8. Simmer for 15 minutes.
9. Put one-half cup of sauce in the bottom of a baking dish.
10. Lay the cutlets in the sauce and top with remaining sauce and mozzarella.
11. Bake for ten minutes.

Meatballs

Meatballs are delicious any way you serve them. These would be great by themselves or on top of some spaghetti squash with your favorite sauce.

Ingredients:

¼ tsp. baking soda

1 tbsp. coconut flour

2 tbsp. Dijon

1 lb. ground beef

2 tbsp. tomato paste

½ tsp. sea salt

Shallot, minced

1 large egg

½ tsp. pepper

Instructions:

1. Your oven needs to be at 350.
2. Add the shallot, beef, and egg to a bowl.
3. Mix well to combine.
4. Stir in the rest of the ingredients.
5. Take a quarter cup of the mixture and form into a ball.
6. Put on a baking sheet.
7. Continue until all meat mixture is used.
8. Bake for 25 minutes until done.

Curried Shrimp

This dish is light but still decadent. It would be great served with a light summer salad and eaten outside while enjoying nature.

Ingredients:

3 tbsp. lime juice

4 tbsp. olive oil

1 lb. shrimp, peeled

4 garlic cloves

Bunch Cilantro, chopped

1 chopped onion

½ tsp. turmeric

½ c pureed tomatoes

½ tsp. coriander

2 tsp. minced ginger

½ tsp. cumin

Instructions:

1. Warm oil in the skillet.
2. Add garlic and onions.
3. Cook until soft.
4. Add the turmeric, coriander, cumin, ginger, and tomatoes.
5. Cook for five minutes.
6. Add shrimp and cook until opaque.
7. Add Cilantro and lime juice.
8. Stir to combine.

Beef Brisket

I love slow cooker meals. They are so easy to make and keeps you from standing over a stove for hours. This can be served with any vegetable you love.

Ingredients:

½ tsp. sea salt

1 ½ lb. brisket

8 carrots, sliced

1 tbsp. onion powder

8 oz. mushrooms, sliced

3 c chicken broth

8 garlic cloves, sliced

1 medium chopped onion

1 tbsp. garlic powder

Instructions:

1. Place carrots on bottom of crock pot.
2. Mix garlic powder, garlic, onion powder, salt, mushrooms, and broth together in a bowl.
3. Put the meat on top of the carrots.
4. Pour broth mixture over top of meat.
5. Cover.
6. Set for six to eight hours on low.

Chicken Piccata

Ingredients:

¼ c parsley

1 ½ lb. chicken breast halves

5 tbsp. olive oil

5 tbsp. grape seed oil

¼ c capers

½ c almond flour

1 c chicken stock

½ tsp. sea salt

¼ c lemon juice

½ tsp. chef's shake

Instructions:

1. Butterfly the chicken and pound to a quarter of an inch thin.
2. Add the chef's shake, flour, and salt to a bowl.
3. Mix to combine.
4. Dredge each piece of chicken in the flour.
5. Warm two tablespoons of grape seed oil and the olive oil in a skillet.
6. Brown the chicken and put them in a warm oven to stay warm.
7. Put capers, lemon juice, and stock into the skillet and deglaze.
8. Reduce heat and add the rest of the grape seed oil.
9. Let cook for a few minutes.
10. Put chicken on a plate and drizzle with the sauce.
11. Sprinkle with parsley.

Chipotle Lime Salmon

Ingredients:

1 tsp. chipotle powder

2 tbsp. olive oil

2 limes, halved

1 lb. salmon, cut into four fillets

1 tsp. sea salt

Instructions:

1. Your oven should be at 500.
2. Rub the fillets with oil.
3. Squeeze each fillet with lime.
4. Sprinkle on chipotle and salt.
5. Reduce temperature to 275.
6. Slide the fillets in the oven and cook 8 to 12 minutes.

Chicken with Cauliflower

This is a quick and easy dish to prepare. Put everything in a pan let it sit and bake it. Nothing is simpler than a one pan meal.

Instructions:

5 garlic cloves, sliced

3 tbsp. olive oil

1 lemon, zested

Bunch thyme

½ tsp. sea salt

1 large head cauliflower, cut into florets

1 c black olives

1 chopped shallot

¼ c lemon juice

1 lb. chicken breast

1 tsp. pepper

Instructions:

1. Your oven needs to be at 400.
2. Place the thyme evenly on the bottom of a baking dish.
3. Put the chicken on top of thyme.
4. Add cauliflower to the top of the chicken.
5. Combine the rest of the ingredients together, and pour over the chicken.
6. Let marinate for an hour.
7. Cook for 45 to 55 minutes.
8. Chicken is done when the internal temperature reaches 165.

Roasted Chicken

Nothing smells better than roasting a chicken. This is a quick and easy way to have a roasted chicken on the table within two hours. Serve with favorite side and have a great meal.

Ingredients:

Onion, quartered

Whole chicken

2 tbsp. olive oil

Salt

Head garlic, cut in half

Pepper

Lemon, halved

Bunch thyme

Instructions:

1. Your oven needs to be set at 425.
2. Clean the chicken and dry completely.
3. Put into a baking dish.
4. Sprinkle liberally with pepper and salt.
5. Put the garlic, lemon, and thyme inside the chicken's cavity.
6. Brush with oil and sprinkle with more pepper and salt.
7. Tie legs down and tuck in the wings.
8. Put one onion quarter in each corner of the baking dish.
9. Cook for an hour and a half.
10. The chicken will be done when internal temperature reaches 165.

Sesame Kelp Noodles

This is an easy way to get a meal on the table in just a matter of minutes. This can be a stand-alone meal or serve it with whatever you would like.

Ingredients:

3 drops stevia

Package kelp noodles

2 tsp. Ume plum vinegar

½ c almond butter

1 tbsp. sesame oil

Instructions:

1. Place the noodles into warm water to soften.
2. Sprinkle with salt.
3. Mix remaining ingredients together.
4. Once noodles are soft, toss with remaining ingredients.
5. Enjoy.

Mustard Lime Chicken

Ingredients:

1 tbsp. olive oil

1 lb. chicken breast

¼ cup Dijon

1 tbsp. chili powder

½ tsp. pepper

½ c chopped Cilantro

½ c lime juice

½ tsp. sea salt

Instructions:

1. Your oven needs to be at 350.
2. Put olive oil, Dijon, chili powder, pepper, lime juice, salt, and Cilantro in food processor.
3. Pulse until well combined.
4. Put the chicken in a baking dish.
5. Pour marinade over chicken and let sit for 15 minutes.
6. Cook for 22 minutes.
7. Chicken is done when internal temperature reaches 165.

Stuffed Peppers

Ingredients:

1 tsp. sea salt

1 tsp. chili powder

1 c Cilantro, chopped

6 to 8 bell peppers

2 tsp. cumin

½ c chopped onion

1 lb. ground turkey

8 oz. diced green chilies

Instructions:

1. Your oven needs to be at 350.
2. Add salt, chili powder, cumin, onion, Cilantro, turkey, and chilies to a bowl.
3. Mix well to combine.
4. Cut the tops off peppers and clean out the seeds and ribs.
5. Put them in a baking dish.
6. Divide the turkey mixture evenly between the peppers.
7. Bake for an hour.

Desserts

Lemon Squares

I love lemon anything. These tasty little squares finish out any meal and satisfy that nagging sweet tooth that many of us have.

Ingredients:

Crust:

3 tbsp. softened butter

1 c almond flour

½ tbsp. lemon zest

¼ c coconut flour

¼ c erythritol

Filling:

5 large eggs, beaten

¾ c lemon juice

½ tbsp. lemon zest

¾ c erythritol

½ c almond milk

1 tbsp. softened butter

Topping:

½ tbsp. butter

¾ c toasted unsweetened coconut chips

2 tbsp. almond flour

Instructions:

Crust:

1. Your oven needs to be at 350.
2. Grease an 8X8 baking dish.
3. To a large bowl add lemon zest, sweetener, coconut flour, and almond flour.
4. Cut butter into flour with a fork or pastry cutter until it resembles sand.

5. Press into bottom of baking dish.
6. Bake 15 minutes until golden brown.
7. Sit to the side and let cool.

Filling:

1. Warm a saucepan and add milk, erythritol, and butter.
2. Stir until sweetener and butter are melted and combined.
3. Add lemon juice.
4. If using fresh, strain to get out seeds and pulp.
5. Whisk in eggs slowly and continue to stir until mixture thickens.
6. Pour filling into crust and bake for 15 minutes.

Topping:

1. Add butter, almond flour, and toasted coconut to food processor and pulse until it looks like coarse sand.
2. Sprinkle over lemon filling and bake until top is crispy.
3. Cool before cutting.
4. Cut into 12 equal and enjoy.

Lemon Meringue Custard

This has the consistency of cake icing and makes for a rich dessert to finish off the most elegant of dinners. You or your guests won't believe that this custard is healthy with a minimal number of calories. The fat in this dessert is all healthy fats that our bodies need.

Ingredients:

For Custard:

2 large egg yolks

Zest of two lemons

½ tsp. lemon extract

1 ½ c heavy whipping cream

½ tsp. vanilla extract

Pinch of salt

½ tsp. xanthan gum

1/3 cup stevia erythritol blend

For Meringue:

1/8 tsp. cream of tartar

2 large room temperature egg whites

1/8 tsp. vanilla extract

1 tbsp. stevia erythritol blend

Instructions:

1. Add lemon zest, salt, xanthan gum, and 1/3 cup sweetener to a saucepan.
2. Mix well to combine.
3. Heat saucepan and whisk in about one tablespoon heavy cream.
4. Keep the heat on low and add remaining cream a couple tablespoons at a time.
5. Whisking completely with each addition.
6. Once all the cream is completely incorporated, whisk in yolks.

7. Raise the heat and continue to stir.
8. When done, take off the burner and stir in ½ tsp. lemon and vanilla extracts.
9. Pour into four 4-ounce oven safe ramekins.
10. Prepare the meringue now, so the custard will still be warm when the meringue is put on top.
11. Add egg whites and cream of tartar to the bowl.
12. Blend with a hand mixer until soft peaks form.
13. Spoon over each custard.
14. Seal the edges with meringue.
15. Using a spoon, make peaks on top.
16. Move the oven rack to sit eight inches from broiler.
17. Turn on broiler.
18. Place ramekins on baking sheet and place under the broiler.
19. Once the meringue is browned, remove from the oven and let cool.
20. Store in the fridge until ready to serve.

Berry Popsicles

This refreshing popsicle will cool you off while supplying you with healthy fats that won't hurt your diet at all.

Ingredients:

½ tsp. vanilla extract

1 c frozen blueberries

1 ½ c canned coconut cream

1 c frozen raspberries

1 c water, divided

1 ½ tsp. liquid stevia, divided

Popsicle sticks and molds

Instructions:

1. Add raspberries, ½ tsp. liquid stevia, and ½ cup water to a small saucepan.
2. Bring to a boil and lower to a simmer until fruit has broken down and slightly reduced.
3. Remove from the heat and blend with either a blender or immersion blender to make smooth.
4. Repeat this process for the blueberries.
5. Set the fruits to the side until ready to use.
6. Combine the coconut cream, vanilla extract, and ½ tsp. liquid stevia in a small bowl.

To assemble

1. Equally, divide the raspberry puree between the six popsicle molds.
2. Put in the freezer for at least one hour.
3. When hard, add the coconut cream mixture to the top of the raspberry mixture.
4. Work quickly, so the raspberries don't melt.

5. Freeze this layer about 30 minutes until just set.
6. Watch closely.
7. This layer needs to be solid enough to hold the sticks but soft enough for the sticks to be inserted.
8. Put one stick in each mold.
9. Make sure to leave part of the stick out of the top.
10. Place back into the freezer until frozen solid.
11. When frozen, add the blueberries to the top and put back into the freezer until completely frozen.
12. Freeze completely.
13. When ready to eat, unmold and enjoy.

Mocha Mousse

If you are a fan of mousse but don't like making it, this recipe helps you accomplish the goal of making a decadent but healthy dessert for your family. It's smooth and creamy and filled with all the healthy fats your body needs.

Ingredients:

Cream Cheese Mixture:

3 tsp. instant coffee powder

8 oz. softened cream cheese

2 tbsp. softened butter

3 tbsp. sour cream

¼ c unsweetened cocoa

1 ½ tsp. vanilla extract

1/3 c granulated Stevia erythritol blend

Whipped Cream Mixture:

½ tsp. vanilla extract

2/3 c heavy whipping cream

1 ½ tsp. granulated stevia erythritol blend

Instructions:

1. Add butter, sour cream, and cream cheese to the bowl.
2. Using a hand mixer, blend until smooth.
3. Add vanilla, coffee, cocoa, and sweetener until completely combined.
4. Set to the side.
5. In a different bowl, beat whipping cream until it forms soft peaks.
6. Add vanilla extract and sweetener.
7. Continue to blend until it forms stiff peaks.
8. Fold one-third of the whipped cream into the cream cheese mixture to lighten it.

9. Do not stir. This will deflate all the air.
10. Fold in the rest of the whipped cream until completely combined.
11. Put mousse into dessert dishes and store in the refrigerator until ready to eat.

Gelatin Rum Shots

Alcohol is forbidden with the keto diet, but in moderation, it can be consumed. This delicious dessert lets you have some rum along with your sweets. Some think this diet restricts you of having the "good" stuff but with moderate, you can still enjoy some of your favorites and still lose weight.

Ingredients:

1 c 80 proof rum

½ tsp. coconut extract

1/3 cup powdered erythritol

1 c water

2 envelopes unflavored gelatin

You will need small individual containers.

Additional toppings:

Unsweetened coconut

Whipped cream

Raspberries

Instructions:

1. Put one half cup water into the saucepan and heat to almost boiling.
2. Add one envelope of gelatin and mix well.
3. Add one-half cup of cool water.
4. Stir to combine.
5. Allow to cool slightly
6. Don't let it get firm.
7. Mix powdered sweetener and coconut extract.
8. Try it to see if you need more sweetener.
9. Add rum and mix well.
10. Pour into containers and place in the fridge for an hour to firm up.
11. These can be served just like they are or add toppings of choice.

Sopapilla Cheesecake

I love cheesecake but couldn't figure out a way to have it with the keto diet. That is until I tried this recipe. You might think pork rinds are weird for a crust, but the saltiness just adds another level of flavor to this decadent dessert.

Ingredients:

2 tsp. vanilla extract

1 tbsp. cinnamon*

2 8 oz. pkg softened cream cheese

1 4 oz. bag pork rinds

2 tbsp. granulated erythritol*

5 large eggs

4 tbsp. melted butter

1 ¼ c water

1/3 c confectioners Swerve

*mix cinnamon and erythritol together

Instructions:

1. Put pork rinds in food processor and pulse until fine powder.
2. Your oven needs to be at 350.
3. Place the pork rinds, water, and 3 eggs into the bowl.
4. Mix to combine.
5. Melt two tablespoons of butter in frying pan.
6. When the butter stops foaming, put a large scoop of batter into the pan.
7. Spread it out into a big pancake shape.
8. When batter begins to bubble around the edges, flip carefully.

9. When both sides are done, remove from the pan and continue until all batter is used.
10. You will have four pieces when finished.
11. Put melted butter in bottom of nine-inch pie pan and brush to cover.
12. Place a piece of the pork rind pancake.
13. Arrange the rest of the pieces until bottom is covered.
14. Keep one piece to be used for topping.
15. Brush pancakes with melted butter and sprinkle generously with cinnamon sugar.
16. Bake about ten minutes.
17. Add vanilla, two eggs, swerve, and cream cheese to a bowl.
18. Using a hand mixer, mix until well combined.
19. Spread this over bottom crust.
20. Cut remaining piece of pork rind pancake into wedges and lay evenly on the top.
21. Sprinkle with the remaining cinnamon sugar.
22. Bake for 20 minutes.
23. Allow to cool before cutting.
24. Cut into 10 even wedges and enjoy.

Conclusion

Thanks for making it through to the end of *The Ketogenic Diet Cookbook*. Let's hope it was informative and able to provide you with all of the tools you need to achieve your goals.

The next step is to try these recipes and start your journey to a new you. It's time to recreate yourself and your life. You will soon find you have more energy, and a brand-new outlook on life. Take time for you and enjoy your new lifestyle.

Finally, if you found this book useful in any way, a review on Amazon is always appreciated!